Vegetarian Salads Cookbook

Be Healthy and Fit With Quick and Delicious Vegetarian Salad Recipes

By
Linda Parker

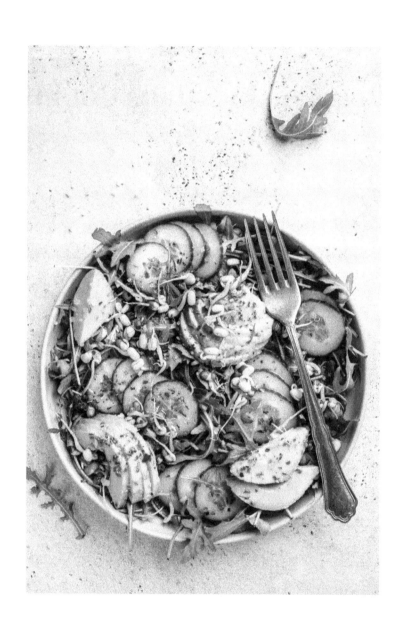

any fashion deemed liable for any hardship or damages that may befall them after undertaking information described herein.

Additionally, the information in the following pages is intended only for informational purposes and should thus be thought of as universal. As befitting its nature, it is presented without assurance regarding its prolonged validity or interim quality. Trademarks that are mentioned are done without written consent and can in no way be considered an endorsement from the trademark holder.

Table of Contents

Introduction   8

Frisee Lettuce and Two-Cheese Salad   11

IceBerg Lettuce and Mozzarella Salad   12

Boston Lettuce and Ricotta Salad   14

Romaine Lettuce Tomatoes and Cream Cheese Salad   15

Stem Lettuce Cucumber and Parmesan Salad   18

Cherry Tomatoes and Pepperjack Cheese Salad   19

Iceberg Lettuce Apples and Mozzarella Salad   21

Frisee Cherries and Parmesan Salad   23

Romaine Lettuce Cherry Tomatoes and Thai Basil Salad   24

Loose-leaf Lettuce Mint Leaves and Cashew Salad   26

Butterhead Lettuce Orange and Monterey Jack Cheese Salad 27

Romaine Lettuce Tomatoes & Pecorino Romano Salad   28

Romaine Lettuce Tomatoes Almond and Tarragon Salad   31

Butter Lettuce and Zucchini with Parmesan Salad   32

Iceberg Lettuce Tomatoes Mozzarella and Almond Salad   33

Romaine Lettuce Cream Cheese and Pistachio Salad   35

Romaine Lettuce with Pepperjack and Feta Salad   36

Frisee Lettuce Tomatoes and Pecorino Romano   38

Boston Lettuce Almond and Vegan Cream Cheese Salad   40

Mesclun and Tomato with Cilantro Vinaigrette   41

Bib Lettuce and Vegan Ricotta Salad   42

Endive Lettuce Tomatillo and Vegan Ricotta Salad   44

Lettuce Tomatillos and Almond Salad   45

Kale Almond and Vegan Ricotta Salad   46

Mesclun Tomatillo and Almond Salad   48

Bib Lettuce Tomatillo and Almond Salad   49

Butter Lettuce and Feta Cheese Salad   50

Mesclun Tomatillo and Cottage Cheese Salad 52

Endive Tomato and Ricotta Cheese Salad 53

Kale Cucumber Tomatillo and Camembert Salad 54

Kale Tomato and Pepper Jack Cheese Salad 55

Napa Cabbage Tomatillo and Tofu Ricotta Cheese Salad 56

Bib Lettuce Tomatillo and Vegan Parmesan Cheese Salad 58

Baby Beet Greens Tomatoes and Tofu Ricotta Cheese Salad 59

Kale and Cheddar Cheese Salad 60

Easy Romaine Lettuce Salad 62

Easy Boston Lettuce and Hazelnut Salad 63

Bibb Lettuce Salad with Balsamic Glaze 64

Mixed Greens Salad 66

Boston Lettuce with Cheddar Cheese and Balsamic Glaze 67

Romaine Lettuce with Feta Cheese 68

Endive with Pepperjack Cheese and Balsamic Vinaigrette Salad 69

Bibb Lettuce with Walnut Vinaigrette Salad 71

Bibb Lettuce with Cheddar Cheese Salad 72

Romaine Lettuce with Pepperjack Cheese Salad 73

Grilled Romaine Lettuce Salad 75

Grilled Romaine Lettuce with Cream Cheese Salad 76

Grilled Boston lettuce and Gouda Cheese Salad 77

Grilled Bib Lettuce and Cream Cheese Salad 79

Grilled Bibb Lettuce and Capers Salad 80

Grilled Bib Lettuce and Kalamata Olives Salad 81

Romaine Lettuce Capers and Almond Vinaigrette 83

Artichoke and Artichoke Hearts with Pecorino Romano 84

Endive with Black Olives and Artichoke Hearts 85

Collard Greens Black Olive and Artichoke Heart Salad 86

Bib Lettuce Black Olives and Artichoke Heart Salad 88

Romaine Lettuce with Artichoke Heart and Cashew Vinaigrette Salad 89

Beetroot Kalamata Olives and Artichoke Heart Salad 90

Boston Lettuce Baby Carrots and Artichoke Heart Salad 91

Romaine Lettuce & Baby Carrots with Walnut Vinaigrette Salad 93

Romaine Lettuce Green Olives and Artichoke Heart with Macadamia Vinaigrette 94

Collard Greens with Baby Corn Salad 95

Bib Lettuce Black Olives and Baby Corn with Almond Vinaigrette Salad 97

Mixed Greens Olives and Artichoke Heart Salad 98

Artichoke Capers and Artichoke Heart Salad 99

Bibb Lettuce with Tomatillo Dressing 100

Plum Tomato Cucumber and Ricotta Salad 102

Introduction

Vegetarianism refers to a lifestyle that excludes the consumption of all forms of meat including pork, chicken, beef, lamb, venison, fish, and shells. Depending on a person's belief and lifestyle, vegetarianism has different spectrums. There are vegetarians, who like to consume products that come from animals such as milk, eggs, cream and cheese. On the other end of that spectrum are the vegans. Vegans never consume meat or any product that comes from animals.

Benefits of Vegetarianism

According to research, living a vegetarian lifestyle lowers your risk of getting some of the major chronic diseases such as heart disease, cancer and type 2 diabetes. Vegetarians are 19 to 25% less likely to die of any kind of heart disease. The high consumption of fiber from grains also prevents the blood sugar spikes that lead to heart attacks and diabetes. The consumption of nuts, which are high in fiber, antioxidants and omega 3 fatty acids also helps lower the vegetarian's risk of getting heart attacks.

Due to the avoidance of red meat, you'll also eliminate a great deal of risk in getting certain types of cancer such as colon cancer. The high level of antioxidants from green leafy vegetables and fruits also helps in this area.

What About These Missing Nutrients?

Some people may be concerned with the lack of the following nutrients in a vegetarian diet however you'll find that there are certain types of vegetables and fruits that can supply these nutrients to give you a perfectly balanced diet. Some of the nutrients of concern are protein, iron, calcium and vitamin b12.

Protein can easily be found in beans and products made from beans such as tofu. Nuts and peas are also good sources of protein. Iron can also be found in tofu, beans, spinach, chard and cashews. Calcium can easily be found in soy milk, broccoli, collard greens, mustard greens and kale.

How to Make The Change

When you're starting out with this lifestyle, you might want to take baby steps. Start with 1 vegetarian meal per day. This allows you to adapt gradually to the different taste and flavors of a vegetarian diet. Once you're used to having a vegetarian meal every day, you can slowly add one more vegetarian meal until you've completely changed your lifestyle. Research has found that making small changes is more sustainable in the end. It's not a contest. Take your time and enjoy the different types of vegetarian meals. How To Use This Book As you browse through the pages, figure out which recipes you like and make them a part of your daily life. This book is filled with different types of vegan dishes and some of them include classic dishes that have been adapted to suit the vegan diet.

Frisee Lettuce and Two-Cheese Salad

Ingredients:

- 3 ounces pecorino romano cheese, shredded
- 3 ounces cheddar cheese , shredded
- 3 ounces monterey jack cheese, shredded
- 8 ounces vegan cheese
- 6 to 7 cups frisee lettuce, 3 bundles, trimmed
- 1/4 European or seedless cucumber, halved lengthwise, then thinly sliced
- 3 tablespoons chopped or snipped chives
- 16 cherry tomatoes
- 1/2 cup sliced almonds
- 1/4 white onion, sliced
- 2 to 3 tablespoons chopped tarragon leaves
- Salt and pepper, to taste

Dressing:

- 1 small shallot, minced
- 1 tablespoon distilled white vinegar
- 1/4 lemon, juiced, about 2 teaspoons
- 1/4 cup extra-virgin olive oil

Directions:

1. Combine all of the dressing ingredients in a food processor.
2. Toss with the rest of the ingredients and combine well.

IceBerg Lettuce and Mozzarella Salad

Ingredients:
- 3 ounces mozzarella cheese, shredded
- 3 ounces cheddar cheese , shredded
- 6 to 7 cups iceberg lettuce,
- 3 bundles, trimmed
- 1/4 seedless cucumber, halved lengthwise, then thinly sliced
- 3 tablespoons chopped or snipped chives
- 16 small tomatoes
- 1/2 cup peanuts
- 1/4 vidalia onion, sliced
- 2 to 3 tablespoons chopped thyme leaves
- Salt and pepper, to taste
- 3 ounces cheddar cheese , shredded
- 3 ounces monterey jack cheese, shredded

Dressing:
- 1 small shallot, minced
- 1 tablespoon distilled white vinegar
- 1/4 lemon, juiced, about 2 teaspoons
- 1/4 cup extra-virgin olive oil
- 1/2 tsp. English mustard Prep

Directions:

1. Combine all of the dressing ingredients in a food processor.
2. Toss with the rest of the ingredients and combine well.

Boston Lettuce and Ricotta Salad

Ingredients:
- 6 to 7 cups Boston lettuce,
- 3 bundles, trimmed
- 1/4 European or seedless cucumber, halved lengthwise, then thinly sliced
- 3 tablespoons chopped or snipped chives
- 16 cherry tomatoes
- 1/2 cup sliced walnuts
- 1/4 red onion, sliced
- 2 to 3 tablespoons chopped tarragon leaves
- Salt and pepper, to taste
- 3 ounces pepper jack cheese, shredded
- 3 ounces ricotta cheese
- 3 ounces cream cheese, crumbled

Dressing:
- 1 small shallot, minced
- 1 tablespoon distilled white vinegar
- 1/4 lemon, juiced, about 2 teaspoons
- 1/4 cup extra-virgin olive oil
- 1 tbsp. egg free mayonnaise Prep

Directions:
1. Combine all of the dressing ingredients in a food processor.
2. Toss with the rest of the ingredients and combine well.

Romaine Lettuce Tomatoes and Cream Cheese Salad

Ingredients:
- 7 cups Romaine lettuce
- 3 bundles, trimmed
- 1/4 European or seedless cucumber, halved lengthwise, then thinly sliced
- 3 tablespoons chopped or snipped chives
- 16 cherry tomatoes
- 1/2 cup sliced walnuts
- 1/4 white onion, sliced
- 2 to 3 tablespoons chopped tarragon leaves
- Salt and pepper, to taste
- 3 ounces ricotta cheese
- 3 ounces cream cheese, crumbled
- 3 ounces parmesan cheese, shredded

Dressing:
- 1 small shallot, minced
- 1 tablespoon distilled white vinegar
- 1/4 lemon, juiced, about 2 teaspoons
- 1/4 cup extra-virgin olive oil
- Egg-free mayonnaise

Directions:

1. Combine all of the dressing ingredients in a food processor.
2. Toss with the rest of the ingredients and combine well.

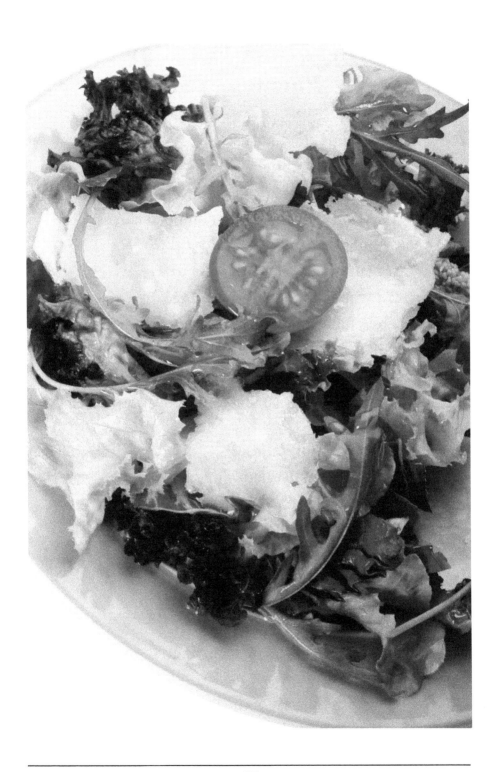

Stem Lettuce Cucumber and Parmesan Salad

Ingredients:

- 6 to 7 cups stem lettuce
- 3 bundles, trimmed
- 1/4 cucumber, halved lengthwise, then thinly sliced
- 3 tablespoons chopped or snipped chives
- 2 mangoes, cubed
- 1/2 cup sliced almonds
- 1/4 white onion, sliced
- 2 to 3 tablespoons chopped tarragon leaves
- Salt and pepper, to taste
- 6 ounces cream cheese, crumbled
- 3 ounces parmesan cheese, shredded

Dressing:

- 1 small shallot, minced
- 1 tablespoon distilled white vinegar
- 1/4 lime, juiced, about 2 teaspoons
- 1/4 cup extra-virgin olive oil
- 1 tbsp. honey
- 1 tsp. English mustard

Directions:

1. Combine all of the dressing ingredients in a food processor.
2. Toss with the rest of the ingredients and combine well.

Cherry Tomatoes and Pepperjack Cheese Salad

Ingredients:
- 7 cups iceberg lettuce
- 3 bundles, trimmed
- 1/4 European or seedless cucumber, halved lengthwise, then thinly sliced
- 3 tablespoons chopped or snipped chives
- 15 cherry tomatoes
- 1/2 cup cashews
- 1/4 white onion, sliced
- 2 to 3 tablespoons chopped tarragon leaves
- Salt and pepper, to taste
- 4 ounces cheddar cheese , shredded
- 3 ounces pepper jack cheese,

Dressing:
- 1 small shallot, minced
- 1 tablespoon distilled white vinegar
- 1/4 lemon, juiced, about 2 teaspoons
- 1/4 cup extra-virgin olive oil

Directions:
1. Combine all of the dressing ingredients in a food processor.
2. Toss with the rest of the ingredients and combine well.

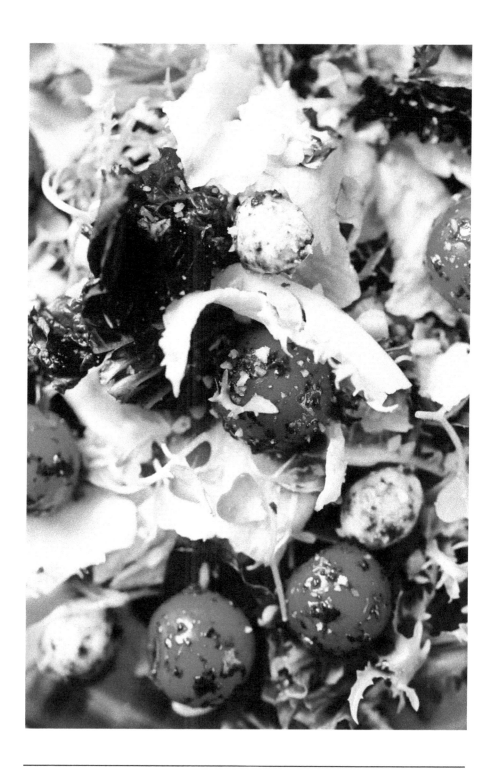

Iceberg Lettuce Apples and Mozzarella Salad

Ingredients:

- 3 ounces mozzarella cheese, shredded
- 3 ounces cheddar cheese , shredded
- 3 ounces pepper jack cheese, shredded
- 6 to 7 cups iceberg lettuce
- 3 bundles, trimmed
- 1/4 European or seedless cucumber, halved lengthwise, then thinly sliced
- 3 tablespoons chopped or snipped chives
- 2 apples, cored and cubed into 2 inch cubes
- 1/2 cup sliced walnuts
- 1/4 white onion, sliced
- 2 to 3 tablespoons chopped tarragon leaves
- Salt and pepper, to taste

Dressing:

- 1 small shallot, minced
- 2 tablespoons distilled white vinegar
- 1/4 cup sesame oil
- 1 teaspoon honey
- 1/2 tsp. egg-free mayonnaise

Directions:

1. Combine all of the dressing ingredients in a food processor.
2. Toss with the rest of the ingredients and combine well.

Frisee Cherries and Parmesan Salad

Ingredients:

- 6 to 7 cups frisee lettuce
- 3 bundles, trimmed
- 1/4 European or seedless cucumber, halved lengthwise, then thinly sliced
- 3 tablespoons chopped or snipped chives
- 16 cherries, pitted
- 1/2 cup macadamia nuts
- 1/4 red onion, sliced
- 2 to 3 tablespoons chopped tarragon leaves
- Sea salt and pepper, to taste
- 3 ounces pepper jack cheese, shredded
- 3 ounces ricotta cheese
- 3 ounces parmesan cheese, shredded

Dressing:

- 1 tbsp. chives, snipped
- 1 tablespoon distilled white vinegar
- 1/4 lemon, juiced, about 2 teaspoons
- 1/4 cup extra-virgin olive oil
- 1 tbsp. honey

Directions:

1. Combine all of the dressing ingredients in a food processor.
2. Toss with the rest of the ingredients and combine well.

Romaine Lettuce Cherry Tomatoes and Thai Basil Salad

Ingredients:

- 6 to 7 cups Romaine lettuce
- 3 bundles, trimmed
- 1/4 European or seedless cucumber, halved lengthwise, then thinly sliced
- 3 tablespoons chopped or snipped chives
- 16 cherry tomatoes
- 1/2 cup walnuts
- 1/4 white onion, sliced
- 2 to 3 tablespoons chopped
- Thai basil Salt and pepper, to taste

Dressing:

- 1 small scallions, minced
- 1 tablespoon distilled white vinegar
- 1/4 cup sesame oil
- 1 tbsp.sambal oelek

Directions:

1. Combine all of the dressing ingredients in a food processor.
2. Toss with the rest of the ingredients and combine well.

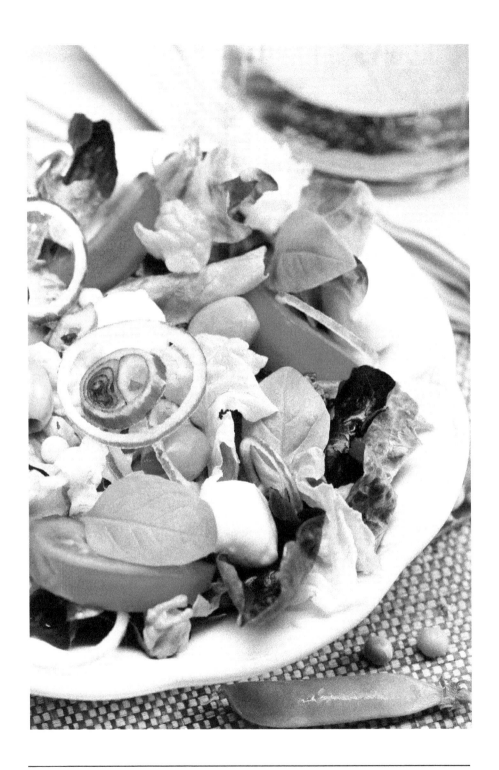

Loose-leaf Lettuce Mint Leaves and Cashew Salad

Ingredients:
- 6 to 7 cups loose leaf lettuce,
- 3 bundles, trimmed
- 1/4 European or seedless cucumber, halved lengthwise, then thinly sliced
- 3 tablespoons chopped or snipped chives 16 grapes
- 1/2 cup cashews
- 1/4 red onion, sliced
- 2 to 3 tablespoons chopped mint leaves
- Salt and pepper, to taste
- 3 ounces pepper jack cheese, shredded
- 3 ounces ricotta cheese
- 3 ounces parmesan cheese, shredded

Dressing:
- 1 small shallot, minced
- 1 tablespoon distilled white vinegar
- 1/4 lime, juiced, about 2 teaspoons
- 1/4 cup extra-virgin olive oil
- 1 tsp. honey

Directions:
1. Combine all of the dressing ingredients in a food processor.
2. Toss with the rest of the ingredients and combine well.

Butterhead Lettuce Orange and Monterey Jack Cheese Salad

Ingredients:
- 6 to 7 cups Butter head lettuce,
- 3 bundles, trimmed
- 1/4 cucumber, halved lengthwise, then thinly sliced
- 3 tablespoons chopped or snipped mint leaves
- 8 slices of mandarin oranges, skins removed and sliced in half 1/2 cup sliced almonds
- 1/4 white onion, sliced
- Salt and pepper, to taste
- 3 ounces pecorino romano cheese, shredded
- 3 ounces cream cheese, crumbled
- 3 ounces monterey jack cheese, shredded

Dressing:
- 1 small shallot, minced 1 tablespoon distilled white vinegar
- 1/4 lime, juiced, about 2 teaspoons
- 1/4 cup sesame oil 1 tbsp. honey

Directions:
1. Combine all of the dressing ingredients in a food processor.
2. Toss with the rest of the ingredients and combine well.

Romaine Lettuce Tomatoes & Pecorino Romano Salad

Ingredients:
- 6 to 7 cups Iceberg lettuce,
- 3 bundles, trimmed
- 1/4 European or seedless cucumber, halved lengthwise, then thinly sliced
- 3 tablespoons chopped or snipped chives
- 16 cherry tomatoes
- 1/2 cup hazelnuts
- 10 black grapes, seedless
- 2 to 3 tablespoons chopped tarragon leaves
- Salt and pepper, to taste
- 6 ounces ricotta cheese
- 1 ounces parmesan cheese, shredded
- 1 ounces pecorino romano cheese, shredded

Dressing:
- 1 small shallot, minced
- 1 tablespoon distilled white vinegar
- 1/4 lemon, juiced, about 2 teaspoons
- 1/4 cup extra-virgin olive oil
- 1 tbsp. honey

Directions:

1. Combine all of the dressing ingredients in a food processor.
2. Toss with the rest of the ingredients and combine well.

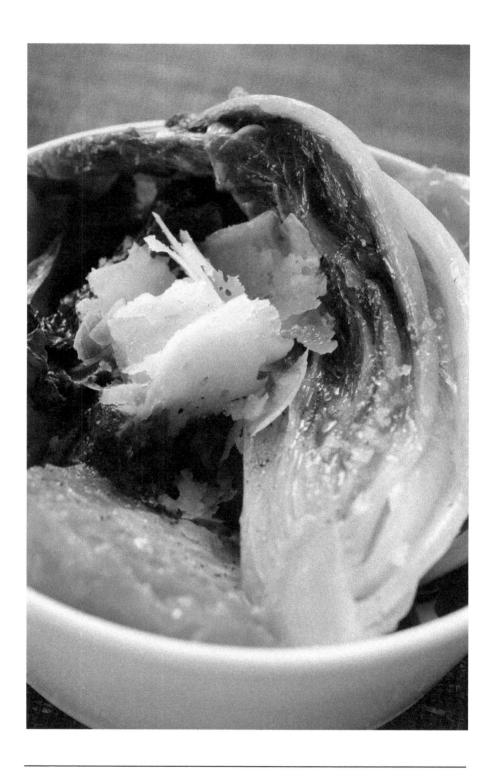

Romaine Lettuce Tomatoes Almond and Tarragon Salad

Ingredients:

- 3 ounces pecorino romano cheese, shredded
- 3 ounces cream cheese, crumbled
- 3 ounces mozzarella cheese, shredded
- 6 to 7 cups Romaine lettuce,
- 3 bundles, trimmed
- 1/4 European or seedless cucumber, halved lengthwise, then thinly sliced
- 3 tablespoons chopped or snipped chives
- 16 cherry tomatoes
- 1/2 cup sliced almonds
- 1/4 white onion, sliced
- 2 to 3 tablespoons chopped tarragon leaves
- Salt and pepper, to taste

Dressing:

- 1 small shallot, minced
- 1 tablespoon distilled white vinegar
- 1/4 lemon, juiced, about 2 teaspoons
- 1/4 cup extra-virgin olive oil

Directions:

1. Combine all of the dressing ingredients in a food processor.
2. Toss with the rest of the ingredients and combine well.

Butter Lettuce and Zucchini with Parmesan Salad

Ingredients:

- 5 ounces cream cheese, crumbled
- 3 ounces mozzarella cheese, shredded
- 1 ounces parmesan cheese, shredded
- 6 to 7 cups Butter lettuce,
- 3 bundles, trimmed
- 1/4 Zucchini, halved lengthwise, then thinly sliced
- 16 cherry tomatoes
- 1/2 cup sliced almonds
- 1/4 white onion, sliced
- 2 to 3 tablespoons chopped tarragon leaves
- Salt and pepper, to taste

Dressing:

- 1 small shallot, minced
- 1 tablespoon distilled white vinegar
- 1/4 lemon, juiced, about 2 teaspoons
- 1/4 cup extra-virgin olive oil

Directions:

1. Combine all of the dressing ingredients in a food processor.
2. Toss with the rest of the ingredients and combine well.

Iceberg Lettuce Tomatoes Mozzarella and Almond Salad

Ingredients:

- 3 ounces cream cheese, crumbled
- 5 ounces mozzarella cheese, shredded
- 6 to 7 cups Iceberg lettuce,
- 3 bundles, trimmed
- 1/4 European or seedless cucumber, halved lengthwise, then thinly sliced
- 3 tablespoons chopped or snipped chives
- 16 cherry tomatoes
- 1/2 cup sliced almonds
- 1/4 white onion, sliced
- 2 to 3 tablespoons chopped tarragon leaves
- Salt and pepper, to taste

Dressing:

- 1 small shallot, minced
- 1 tablespoon distilled white vinegar
- 1/4 lemon, juiced, about 2 teaspoons
- 1/4 cup extra-virgin olive oil

Directions:

1. Combine all of the dressing ingredients in a food processor.
2. Toss with the rest of the ingredients and combine well.

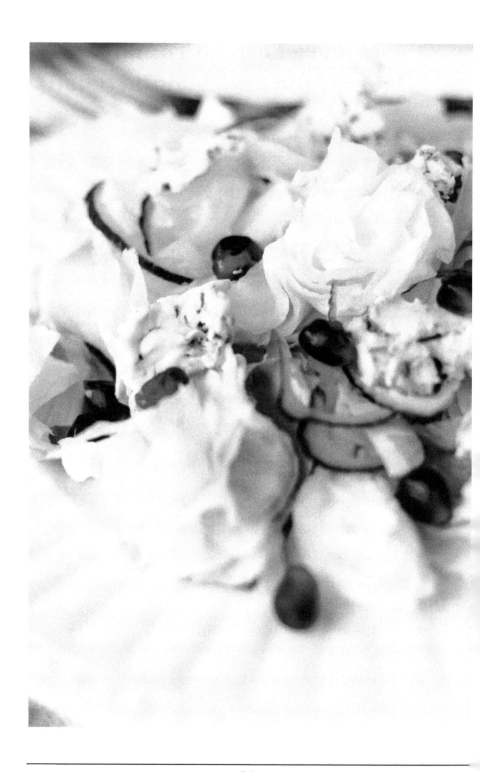

Romaine Lettuce Cream Cheese and Pistachio Salad

Ingredients:
- 5 ounces cream cheese, crumbled
- 3 ounces mozzarella cheese, shredded
- 6 to 7 cups Romaine lettuce,
- 3 bundles, trimmed
- 1/4 European or seedless cucumber, halved lengthwise, then thinly sliced
- 3 tablespoons chopped or snipped chives
- 16 cherry tomatoes
- 1/2 cup sliced pistachios
- 1/4 Vidalia onion, sliced
- 2 to 3 tablespoons chopped tarragon leaves
- Salt and pepper, to taste

Dressing:
- 1 small shallot, minced
- 1 tablespoon distilled white vinegar
- 1/4 lemon, juiced, about 2 teaspoons
- 1/4 cup extra-virgin olive oil

Directions:
1. Combine all of the dressing ingredients in a food processor.
2. Toss with the rest of the ingredients and combine well.

Romaine Lettuce with Pepperjack and Feta Salad

Ingredients:
- 6 to 7 cups romaine lettuce
- 3 bundles, trimmed
- 1/4 European or seedless cucumber, halved lengthwise, then thinly sliced
- 3 tablespoons chopped or snipped chives
- 16 cherry tomatoes
- 1/2 cup macadamia nuts
- 1/4 red onion, sliced
- Salt and pepper, to taste
- 1 ounces monterey jack cheese, shredded
- 3 ounces ricotta cheese
- 1 ounces cheddar cheese , shredded
- 1 ounces pepper jack cheese, shredded

Dressing:
- 1 small shallot, minced
- 1 tablespoon distilled white vinegar
- 1/4 lemon, juiced, about 2 teaspoons
- 1/4 cup extra-virgin olive oil
- 1 tbsp. pesto sauce

Directions:

1. Combine all of the dressing ingredients in a food processor.
2. Toss with the rest of the ingredients and combine well.

Frisee Lettuce Tomatoes and Pecorino Romano

Ingredients:
- 6 to 7 cups frisee lettuce
- 3 bundles, trimmed
- 1/4 cucumber, halved lengthwise, then thinly sliced
- 3 tablespoons chopped or snipped chives
- 16 cherry tomatoes
- 1/2 cup sliced almonds
- 1/4 red onion, sliced
- 2 to 3 tablespoons chopped parsley
- Salt and pepper, to taste
- 3 ounces ricotta cheese
- 2 ounces cheddar cheese , shredded
- 1 ounces pepper jack cheese, shredded
- 1 ounces pecorino romano cheese, shredded

Dressing:
- 1 small scallions, minced
- 1 tablespoon distilled white vinegar
- 1/4 lemon, juiced, about 2 teaspoons
- 1/4 cup macadamia nut oil

Directions:
1. Combine all of the dressing ingredients in a food processor.
2. Toss with the rest of the ingredients and combine well.

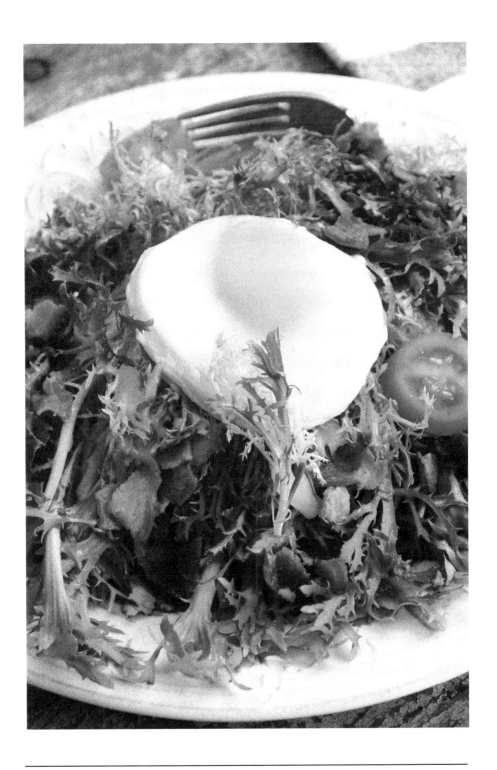

Boston Lettuce Almond and Vegan Cream Cheese Salad

Ingredients:
- 7 cups Boston lettuce
- 3 bundles, trimmed
- 1/2 cucumber, halved lengthwise, then thinly sliced
- 3 tablespoons chopped or snipped chives
- 16 cherry tomatoes
- 1/2 cup sliced almonds
- 1/4 red onion, sliced
- Salt and pepper, to taste
- 7 ounces vegan cream cheese

Dressing:
- 1 small shallot, minced
- 1 tablespoon distilled white vinegar
- 1/4 lemon, juiced, about 2 teaspoons
- 1/4 cup extra-virgin olive oil
- 1 tbsp. chimichurri sauce

Directions:
1. Combine all of the dressing ingredients in a food processor.
2. Toss with the rest of the ingredients and combine well.

Mesclun and Tomato with Cilantro Vinaigrette

Ingredients:

- 6 to 7 cups mesclun,
- 3 bundles, trimmed
- 1/4 cucumber, halved lengthwise, then thinly sliced
- 3 tablespoons chopped or snipped chives
- 16 cherry tomatoes
- 1/2 cup sliced almonds
- 1/4 white onion, sliced
- Salt and pepper, to taste
- 1 ounce blue cheese, crumbled
- 3 ounces gouda cheese, shredded
- 3 ounces brie cheese, crumbled

Dressing:

- 1 sprig cilantro, minced
- 1 tablespoon distilled white vinegar
- 1/4 lemon, juiced, about 2 teaspoons
- 1/4 cup extra-virgin olive oil

Directions:

1. Combine all of the dressing ingredients in a food processor.
2. Toss with the rest of the ingredients and combine well.

Bib Lettuce and Vegan Ricotta Salad

Ingredients:

- 6 to 7 cups bib lettuce
- 3 bundles, trimmed
- 1/4 cucumber, halved lengthwise, then thinly sliced
- 16 grapes
- 1/2 cup sliced almonds
- 1/4 white onion, sliced
- Salt and pepper, to taste
- 3 ounces mozzarella cheese, shredded
- 3 ounces parmesan cheese, shredded
- 1 ounce blue cheese, crumbled

Dressing:

- **1 t**ablespoon distilled white vinegar
- 1/4 lemon, juiced, about 2 teaspoons
- 1/4 cup extra-virgin olive oil
- 1 tbsp. Chimichurri sauce

Directions:

1. Combine all of the dressing ingredients in a food processor.
2. Toss with the rest of the ingredients and combine well.

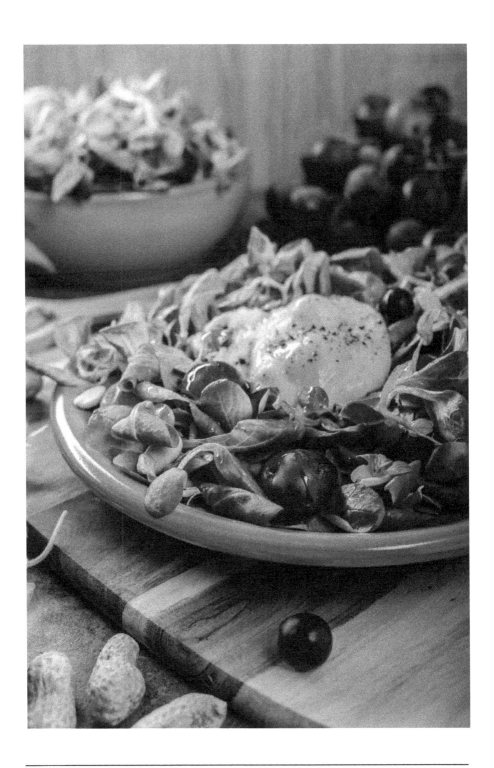

Endive Lettuce Tomatillo and Vegan Ricotta Salad

Ingredients:
- 6 to 7 cups endive,
- 3 bundles, trimmed
- 1/4 cucumber, halved lengthwise, then thinly sliced
- 3 tablespoons chopped or snipped chives
- 16 green tomatillos, sliced in half
- 1/2 cup sliced almonds
- 1/4 white onion, sliced
- Salt and pepper, to taste
- 3 ounces pecorino romano cheese, shredded
- 3 ounces cream cheese, crumbled
- 3 ounces camembert cheese, crumbled

Dressing:
- 1 tablespoon distilled white vinegar
- 1/4 lemon, juiced, about 2 teaspoons
- 1/4 cup extra-virgin olive oil
- 1 tsp. Dijon mustard

Directions:
1. Combine all of the dressing ingredients in a food processor.
2. Toss with the rest of the ingredients and combine well.

Lettuce Tomatillos and Almond Salad

Ingredients:
- 6 to 7 cups lettuce
- 3 bundles, trimmed
- 1/4 cucumber, halved lengthwise, then thinly sliced
- 3 tablespoons chopped or snipped chives
- 16 tomatillos, sliced in half
- 1/2 cup sliced almonds
- 1/4 white onion, sliced
- Salt and pepper, to taste
- 3 ounces cream cheese, crumbled
- 3 ounces camembert cheese, crumbled
- 3 ounces mozzarella cheese, shredded

Dressing:
- 1 sprig cilantro, minced
- 1 tablespoon distilled white vinegar
- 1/4 lemon, juiced, about 2 teaspoons
- 1/4 cup extra-virgin olive oil
- 1 tsp. English mustard

Directions:
1. Combine all of the dressing ingredients in a food processor.
2. Toss with the rest of the ingredients and combine well.

Kale Almond and Vegan Ricotta Salad

Ingredients:
- 6 to 7 cups kale,
- 3 bundles, trimmed
- 1/4 cucumber, halved lengthwise, then thinly sliced
- 3 tablespoons chopped or snipped chives
- 16 green tomatillos, sliced in half
- 1/2 cup sliced almonds
- 1/4 white onion, sliced
- Salt and pepper, to taste
- 3 ounces cottage cheese, crumbled
- 3 ounces pepper jack cheese, shredded
- 3 ounces pecorino romano cheese, shredded

Dressing:
- 1 tablespoon distilled white vinegar
- 1/4 lemon, juiced, about 2 teaspoons
- 1/4 cup extra-virgin olive oil
- 1 tsp. Dijon mustard

Directions:
1. Combine all of the dressing ingredients in a food processor.
2. Toss with the rest of the ingredients and combine well.

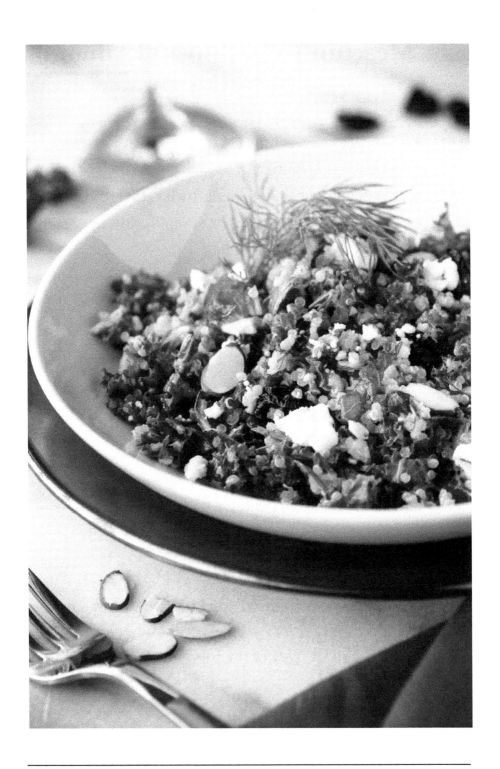

Mesclun Tomatillo and Almond Salad

Ingredients:

- 6 to 7 cups mesclun,
- 3 bundles, trimmed
- 1/4 cucumber, halved lengthwise, then thinly sliced
- 3 tablespoons chopped or snipped chives
- 16 tomatillos, sliced in half
- 1/2 cup sliced almonds
- 1/4 white onion, sliced
- Salt and pepper, to taste
- 3 ounces feta cheese, crumbled
- 3 ounces ricotta cheese
- 3 ounces cheddar cheese , shredded

Dressing:

- 1 tablespoon distilled white vinegar
- 1/4 lemon, juiced, about 2 teaspoons
- 1/4 cup extra-virgin olive oil
- 1 tsp. egg-free mayonnaise

Directions:

1. Combine all of the dressing ingredients in a food processor.
2. Toss with the rest of the ingredients and combine well.

Bib Lettuce Tomatillo and Almond Salad

Ingredients:
- 6 to 7 cups bib lettuce,
- 3 bundles, trimmed
- 1/4 cucumber, halved lengthwise, then thinly sliced
- 3 tablespoons chopped or snipped chives
- 16 tomatillos, sliced in half
- 1/2 cup sliced almonds
- 1/4 white onion, sliced
- Salt and pepper, to taste
- 3 ounces monterey jack cheese, shredded
- 3 ounces feta cheese, crumbled
- 3 ounces ricotta cheese

Dressing:
- 1 tablespoon distilled white vinegar
- 1/4 lemon, juiced, about 2 teaspoons
- 1/4 cup extra-virgin olive oil
- 1 tsp. Dijon mustard

Directions:
1. Combine all of the dressing ingredients in a food processor.
2. Toss with the rest of the ingredients and combine well.

Butter Lettuce and Feta Cheese Salad

Ingredients:
- 6 to 7 cups butter lettuce,
- 3 bundles, trimmed
- 1/4 cucumber, halved lengthwise, then thinly sliced
- 3 tablespoons chopped or snipped chives
- 16 tomatillos, sliced in half
- 1/2 cup sliced almonds
- 1/4 white onion, sliced
- Salt and pepper, to taste
- 6 ounces monterey jack cheese, shredded
- 3 ounces feta cheese, crumbled

Dressing:
- 1 sprig cilantro, minced
- 1 tablespoon distilled white vinegar
- 1/4 lemon, juiced, about 2 teaspoons
- 1/4 cup extra-virgin olive oil
- 1 tsp. egg free mayonnaise

Directions:
1. Combine all of the dressing ingredients in a food processor.
2. Toss with the rest of the ingredients and combine well.

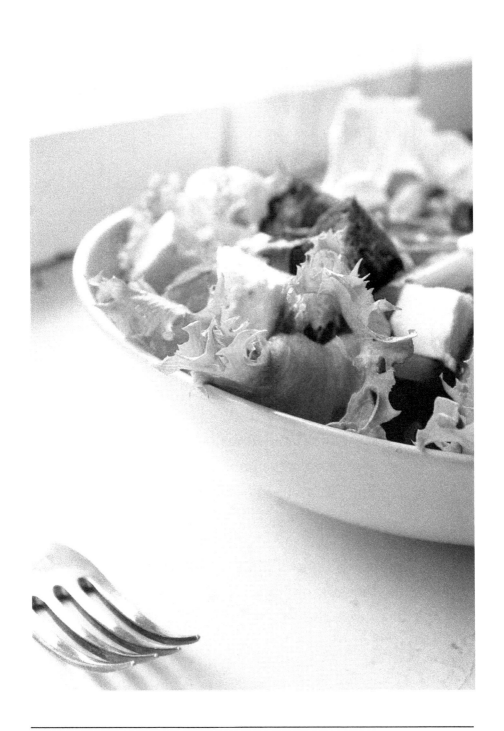

Mesclun Tomatillo and Cottage Cheese Salad

Ingredients:
- 6 to 7 cups mesclun
- 3 bundles, trimmed
- 1/4 cucumber, halved lengthwise, then thinly sliced
- 3 tablespoons chopped or snipped chives
- 16 green tomatillos, sliced in half
- 1/2 cup sliced almonds
- 1/4 white onion, sliced
- Salt and pepper, to taste
- 5 ounces cottage cheese, crumbled
- 3 ounces pepper jack cheese, shredded

Dressing:
- 1 sprig cilantro, minced
- 1 tablespoon distilled white vinegar
- 1/4 lemon, juiced, about 2 teaspoons
- 1/4 cup extra-virgin olive oil

Directions:
1. Prep Combine all of the dressing ingredients in a food processor.
2. Toss with the rest of the ingredients and combine well.

Endive Tomato and Ricotta Cheese Salad

Ingredients:
- 6 to 7 cups endive
- 3 bundles, trimmed
- 1/4 cucumber, halved lengthwise, then thinly sliced
- 3 tablespoons chopped or snipped chives
- 16 cherry tomatoes
- 1/2 cup sliced almonds
- 1/4 white onion, sliced
- Salt and pepper, to taste
- 5 ounces ricotta cheese
- 3 ounces cheddar cheese , shredded

Dressing:
- 1 sprig cilantro, minced
- 1 tablespoon distilled white vinegar
- 1/4 lemon, juiced, about 2 teaspoons
- 1/4 cup extra-virgin olive oil
- 1 tsp. egg free mayonnaise

Directions:
1. Prep Combine all of the dressing ingredients in a food processor.
2. Toss with the rest of the ingredients and combine well.

Kale Cucumber Tomatillo and Camembert Salad

Ingredients:
- 6 to 7 cups kale,
- 3 bundles, trimmed
- 1/4 cucumber, halved lengthwise, then thinly sliced
- 3 tablespoons chopped or snipped chives
- 16 green tomatillos, sliced in half
- 1/2 cup sliced almonds
- 1/4 white onion, sliced
- Salt and pepper, to taste
- 3 ounces cream cheese, crumbled
- 3 ounces camembert cheese, crumbled

Dressing:
- 1 sprig cilantro, minced
- 1 tablespoon distilled white vinegar
- 1/4 lemon, juiced, about 2 teaspoons
- 1/4 cup extra-virgin olive oil
- 1 tsp. English mustard

Directions:
1. Combine all of the dressing ingredients in a food processor.
2. Toss with the rest of the ingredients and combine well.

Kale Tomato and Pepper Jack Cheese Salad

Ingredients:
- 6 to 7 cups kale
- 3 bundles, trimmed
- 1/4 cucumber, halved lengthwise, then thinly sliced
- 3 tablespoons chopped or snipped chives
- 16 cherry tomatoes
- 1/2 cup sliced almonds
- 1/4 white onion, sliced
- Salt and pepper, to taste
- 3 ounces pepper jack cheese, shredded
- 3 ounces pecorino romano cheese, shredded

Dressing:
- 1 sprig cilantro, minced
- 1 tablespoon distilled white vinegar
- 1/4 lemon, juiced, about 2 teaspoons
- 1/4 cup extra-virgin olive oil
- 1 tsp.English mustard

Directions:
1. Combine all of the dressing ingredients in a food processor.
2. Toss with the rest of the ingredients and combine well.

Napa Cabbage Tomatillo and Tofu Ricotta Cheese Salad

Ingredients:
- 6 to 7 cups napa cabbage
- 3 bundles, trimmed
- 1/4 cucumber, halved lengthwise, then thinly sliced
- 3 tablespoons chopped or snipped chives
- 16 green tomatillos, sliced in half
- 1/2 cup sliced almonds
- 1/4 white onion, sliced
- Salt and pepper, to taste
- 1 ounce blue cheese, crumbled
- 6 ounces gouda cheese, shredded

Dressing:
- 1 sprig cilantro, minced
- 1 tablespoon distilled white vinegar
- 1/4 lemon, juiced, about 2 teaspoons
- 1/4 cup extra-virgin olive oil
- 1 tsp. egg free mayonnaise

Directions:
1. Prep Combine all of the dressing ingredients in a food processor.
2. Toss with the rest of the ingredients and combine well.

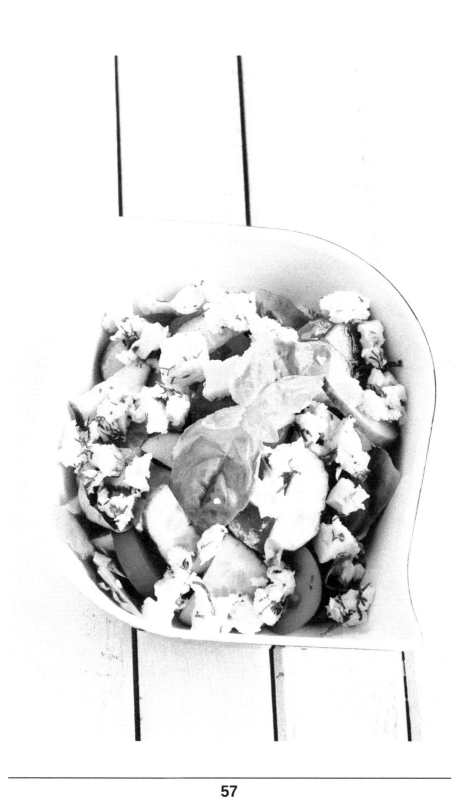

Bib Lettuce Tomatillo and Vegan Parmesan Cheese Salad

Ingredients:
- 6 to 7 cups bib lettuce,
- 3 bundles, trimmed
- 1/4 cucumber, halved lengthwise, then thinly sliced
- 3 tablespoons chopped or snipped chives
- 16 tomatillos, sliced in half
- 1/2 cup sliced almonds
- 1/4 white onion, sliced
- Salt and pepper, to taste
- 7 ounces parmesan cheese, shredded
- 1 ounce blue cheese, crumbled

Dressing:
- 1 sprig cilantro, minced
- 1 tablespoon distilled white vinegar
- 1/4 lemon, juiced, about
- 2 teaspoons
- 1/4 cup extra-virgin olive oil

Directions:
1. Combine all of the dressing ingredients in a food processor.
2. Toss with the rest of the ingredients and combine well.

Baby Beet Greens Tomatoes and Tofu Ricotta Cheese Salad

Ingredients:

- 6 to 7 cups baby beet greens
- 3 bundles, trimmed
- 1/4 cucumber, halved lengthwise, then thinly sliced
- 3 tablespoons chopped or snipped chives
- 16 cherry tomatoes
- 1/2 cup sliced almonds
- 1/4 white onion, sliced
- Salt and pepper, to taste
- 3 ounces cheddar cheese , shredded
- 5 ounces cottage cheese, crumbled

Dressing:

- 1 sprig cilantro, minced
- 1 tablespoon distilled white vinegar
- 1/4 lemon, juiced, about 2 teaspoons
- 1/4 cup extra-virgin olive oil
- 1 tsp. egg free mayonnaise

Directions:

1. Prep Combine all of the dressing ingredients in a food processor.
2. Toss with the rest of the ingredients and combine well.

Kale and Cheddar Cheese Salad

Ingredients:

- 6 to 7 cups kale
- 3 bundles, trimmed
- 1/4 cucumber, halved lengthwise, then thinly sliced
- 3 tablespoons chopped or snipped chives
- 16 tomatillos, sliced in half
- 1/2 cup sliced almonds
- 1/4 white onion, sliced
- Salt and pepper, to taste
- 5 ounces monterey jack cheese, shredded
- 3 ounces cheddar cheese , shredded

Dressing:

- 1 sprig cilantro, minced
- 1 tablespoon distilled white vinegar
- 1/4 lemon, juiced, about 2 teaspoons
- 1/4 cup extra-virgin olive oil
- 1 tsp.English mustard

Directions:

1. Prep Combine all of the dressing ingredients in a food processor.
2. Toss with the rest of the ingredients and combine well.

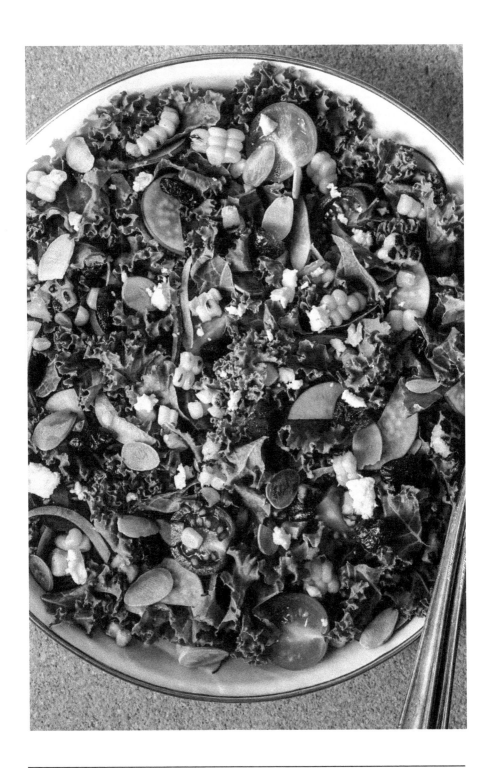

Easy Romaine Lettuce Salad

Ingredients:

- 1 head romaine lettuce, rinsed, patted and shredded

Dressing:

- 2 tbsp. white wine vinegar
- 4 tablespoons macadamia oil
- Freshly ground black pepper
- 3/4 cup finely ground peanuts
- Sea salt

Directions:

1. Prep Combine all of the dressing ingredients in a food processor.
2. Toss with the rest of the ingredients and combine well.

Easy Boston Lettuce and Hazelnut Salad

Ingredients:
- Handful of Boston Lettuce, rinsed, patted and shredded

Dressing:
- 2 tbsp. apple cider vinegar
- 4 tablespoons olive oil
- Freshly ground black pepper
- 3/4 cup finely coarsely ground hazelnuts
- Sea salt

Directions:
1. Combine all of the dressing ingredients in a food processor.
2. Toss with the rest of the ingredients and combine well.

Bibb Lettuce Salad with Balsamic Glaze

Ingredients:
- 1 head bib lettuce, rinsed, patted and shredded

Dressing:
- 2 tbsp. balsamic vinegar
- 4 tablespoons macadamia oil Freshly ground black pepper
- 3/4 cup finely ground almonds Sea salt

Directions:
1. Combine all of the dressing ingredients in a food processor.
2. Toss with the rest of the ingredients and combine well.

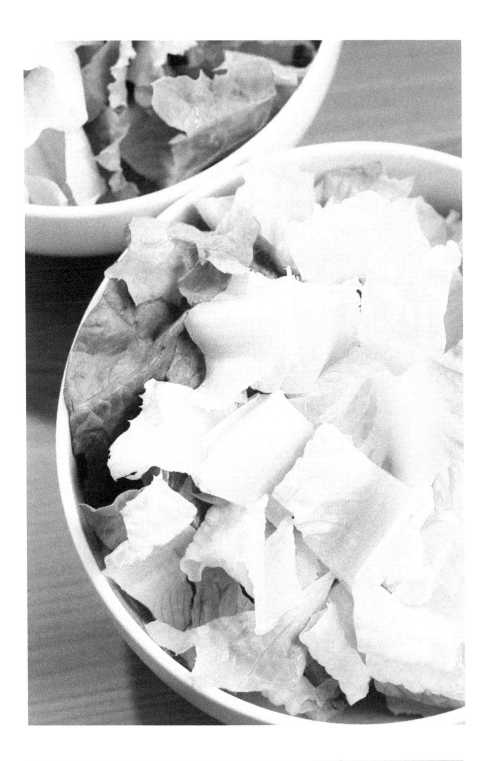

Mixed Greens Salad

Ingredients:
- Handful of Mesclun, rinsed, patted and shredded

Dressing:
- 2 tbsp. distilled white vinegar
- 4 tablespoons extra virgin olive oil
- Freshly ground black pepper
- 3/4 cup finely coarsely ground cashews
- Sea salt

Directions:
1. Combine all of the dressing ingredients in a food processor.
2. Toss with the rest of the ingredients and combine well.

Boston Lettuce with Cheddar Cheese and Balsamic Glaze

Ingredients:
- 1 head Boston lettuce, rinsed, patted and shredded

Dressing:
- 2 tbsp. balsamic vinegar
- 4 tablespoons macadamia oil
- Freshly ground black pepper
- 6 ounces cheddar cheese , shredded
- Sea salt

Directions:
1. Combine all of the dressing ingredients in a food processor.
2. Toss with the rest of the ingredients and combine well.

Romaine Lettuce with Feta Cheese

Ingredients:
- 1 head romaine lettuce, rinsed, patted and shredded

Dressing:
- 2 tbsp. apple cider vinegar
- 4 tablespoons extra virgin olive oil
- Freshly ground black pepper
- 5 ounces feta cheese, crumbled
- Sea salt
-

Directions:
1. Combine all of the dressing ingredients in a food processor.
2. Toss with the rest of the ingredients and combine well.

Endive with Pepperjack Cheese and Balsamic Vinaigrette Salad

Ingredients:

- 1 Head of Endive, rinsed, patted and shredded

Dressing:

- 2 tbsp. balsamic vinegar
- 4 tablespoons extra virgin olive oil
- Freshly ground black pepper
- 4 ounces pepper jack cheese, shredded
- Sea salt

Directions:

1. Combine all of the dressing ingredients in a food processor.
2. Toss with the rest of the ingredients and combine well.

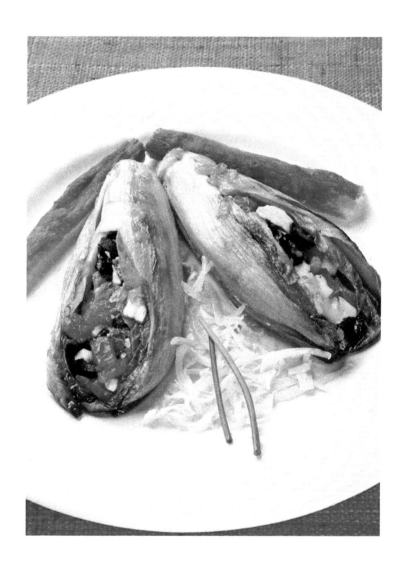

Bibb Lettuce with Walnut Vinaigrette Salad

Ingredients:
- 1 head bib lettuce, rinsed, patted and shredded

Dressing:
- 2 tbsp. red wine vinegar
- 1 tablespoon extra virgin olive oil
- Freshly ground black pepper
- 3/4 cup finely coarsely ground walnuts
- Sea salt

Directions:
1. Combine all of the dressing ingredients in a food processor.
2. Toss with the rest of the ingredients and combine well.

Bibb Lettuce with Cheddar Cheese Salad

Ingredients:
- 1 head bib lettuce, rinsed, patted and shredded

Dressing:
- 2 tbsp. apple cider vinegar
- 4 tablespoons olive oil
- Freshly ground black pepper
- 3 ounces cheddar cheese , shredded
- Sea salt

Directions:
1. Combine all of the dressing ingredients in a food processor.
2. Toss with the rest of the ingredients and combine well.

Romaine Lettuce with Pepperjack Cheese Salad

Ingredients:
- 1 head romaine lettuce, rinsed, patted and shredded

Dressing:
- 2 tbsp. distilled white vinegar
- 4 tablespoons macadamia oil
- Freshly ground black pepper
- 3 ounces pepper jack cheese, shredded
- Sea salt

Directions:
1. Combine all of the dressing ingredients in a food processor.
2. Toss with the rest of the ingredients and combine well.

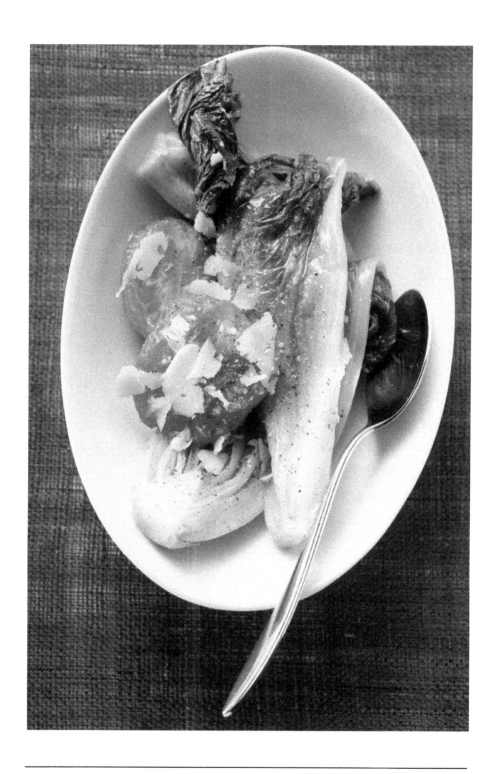

Grilled Romaine Lettuce Salad

Ingredients:
- 1 head romaine lettuce, rinsed, patted and shredded

Dressing:
- 2 tbsp. balsamic vinegar
- 4 tablespoons extra virgin olive oil
- Freshly ground black pepper
- 5 ounces gouda cheese, shredded
- Sea salt
- Grill the lettuce and/or greens over medium heat until lightly charred

Directions:
1. Combine all of the dressing ingredients in a food processor.
2. Toss with the rest of the ingredients and combine well.

Grilled Romaine Lettuce with Cream Cheese Salad

Ingredients:
- 1 head romaine lettuce, rinsed, patted and shredded

Dressing:
- 2 tbsp. red wine vinegar
- 4 tablespoons extra virgin olive oil
- Freshly ground black pepper
- 5 ounces cream cheese, crumbled
- Sea salt
- Grill the lettuce and/or greens over medium heat until lightly charred

Directions:
1. Combine all of the dressing ingredients in a food processor.
2. Toss with the rest of the ingredients and combine well.

Grilled Boston lettuce and Gouda Cheese Salad

Ingredients:
- 1 head Boston lettuce, rinsed, patted and shredded
- 1/2 cup green olives

Dressing:
- 2 tbsp. white wine vinegar
- 4 tablespoons extra virgin olive oil
- Freshly ground black pepper
- 5 ounces gouda cheese, shredded
- Sea salt
- Grill the lettuce and/or greens over medium heat until lightly charred

Directions:
1. Combine all of the dressing ingredients in a food processor.
2. Toss with the rest of the ingredients and combine well.

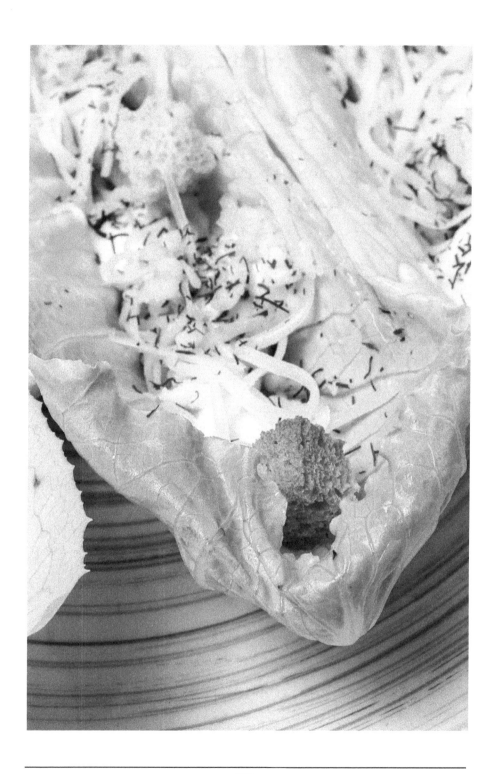

Grilled Bib Lettuce and Cream Cheese Salad

Ingredients:
- 1 head bib lettuce, rinsed, patted and shredded
- 1/2 cup green olives
- 5 ounces cream cheese, crumbled

Dressing:
- 2 tbsp. red wine vinegar
- 4 tablespoons extra virgin olive oil
- Freshly ground black pepper
- 3/4 cup finely ground almonds
- Sea salt
- Grill the lettuce and/or greens over medium heat until lightly charred

Directions:
1. Combine all of the dressing ingredients in a food processor.
2. Toss with the rest of the ingredients and combine well.

Grilled Bibb Lettuce and Capers Salad

Ingredients:
- 1 head bib lettuce, rinsed, patted and shredded
- 1/2cup green capers

Dressing:
- 2 tbsp. white wine vinegar
- 4 tablespoons extra virgin olive oil
- Freshly ground black pepper
- 3/4 cup finely coarsely ground walnuts
- Sea salt
- Grill the lettuce and/or greens over medium heat until lightly charred

Directions:
1. Combine all of the dressing ingredients in a food processor.
2. Toss with the rest of the ingredients and combine well.

Grilled Bib Lettuce and Kalamata Olives Salad

Ingredients:
- 1 head bib lettuce, rinsed, patted and shredded
- 1/2 cup Kalamata olives
- 5 ounces gouda cheese, shredded

Dressing:
- 2 tbsp. red wine vinegar
- 4 tablespoons olive oil
- Freshly ground black pepper
- 3/4 cup finely ground almonds
- Sea salt
- Grill the lettuce and/or greens over medium heat until lightly charred

Directions:
1. Combine all of the dressing ingredients in a food processor.
2. Toss with the rest of the ingredients and combine well.

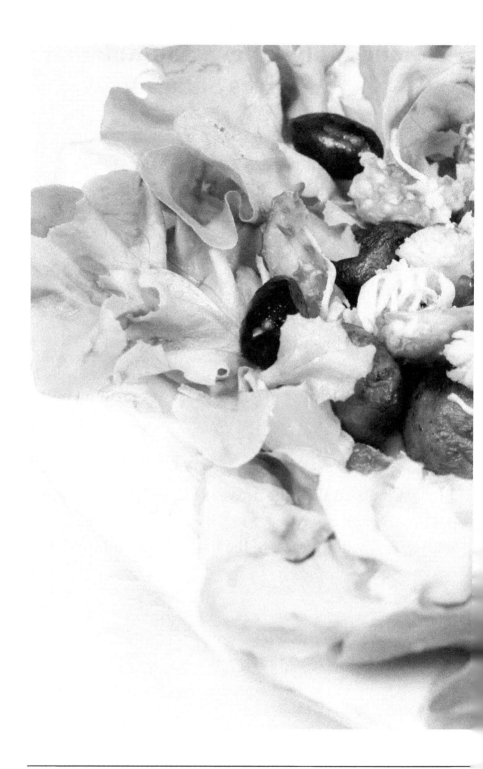

Romaine Lettuce Capers and Almond Vinaigrette

Ingredients:
- 1 head romaine lettuce, rinsed, patted and shredded
- 1/2 cup capers
- 5 ounces ricotta cheese

Dressing:
- 2 tbsp. apple cider vinegar
- 4 tablespoons extra virgin olive oil
- Freshly ground black pepper
- 3/4 cup finely ground almonds
- Sea salt

Directions:
1. Combine all of the dressing ingredients in a food processor.
2. Toss with the rest of the ingredients and combine well.

Artichoke and Artichoke Hearts with Pecorino Romano

Ingredients:
- 1 artichoke, rinsed and patted
- 1/2 cup artichoke hearts
- 5 ounces pecorino romano cheese, shredded

Dressing:
- 2 tbsp. balsamic vinegar
- 4 tablespoons macadamia oil
- Freshly ground black pepper
- 3/4 cup finely ground peanuts
- Sea salt

Directions:
1. Combine all of the dressing ingredients in a food processor.
2. Toss with the rest of the ingredients and combine well.

Endive with Black Olives and Artichoke Hearts

Ingredients:
- 1 head Endive, rinsed, patted and shredded
- 1/2 cup black olives
- 1/2 cup artichoke hearts

Dressing:
- 2 tbsp. apple cider vinegar
- 4 tablespoons olive oil
- Freshly ground black pepper
- 3/4 cup finely ground almonds
- Sea salt

Directions:
1. Combine all of the dressing ingredients in a food processor.
2. Toss with the rest of the ingredients and combine well.

Collard Greens Black Olive and Artichoke Heart Salad

Ingredients:
- 1 bunch collard greens, rinsed, patted and shredded
- 1/2 cup black olives
- 1/2 cup artichoke hearts

Dressing:
- 2 tbsp. red wine vinegar
- 4 tablespoons extra virgin olive oil
- Freshly ground black pepper
- 3/4 cup finely ground almonds Sea salt

Directions:
1. Combine all of the dressing ingredients in a food processor.
2. Toss with the rest of the ingredients and combine well.

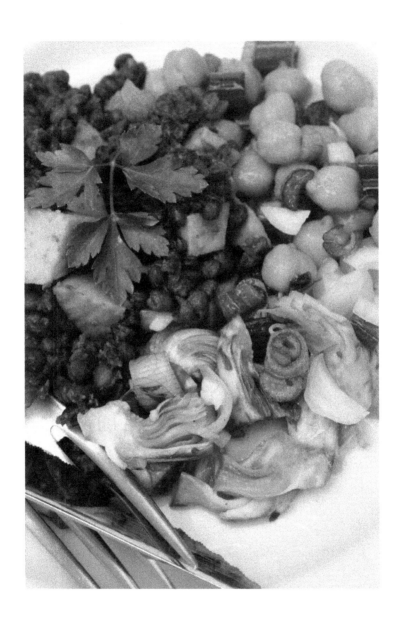

Bib Lettuce Black Olives and Artichoke Heart Salad

Ingredients:
- 1 head bib lettuce, rinsed, patted and shredded
- 1/2 cup black olives
- 1/2 cup artichoke hearts

Dressing:
- 2 tbsp. white wine vinegar
- 4 tablespoons extra virgin olive oil
- Freshly ground black pepper
- 3/4 cup finely ground almonds
- Sea salt

Directions:
1. Combine all of the dressing ingredients in a food processor.
2. Toss with the rest of the ingredients and combine well.

Romaine Lettuce with Artichoke Heart and Cashew Vinaigrette Salad

Ingredients:
- 1 head romaine lettuce, rinsed, patted and shredded
- 1/2 cup black olives
- 1/2 cup artichoke hearts

Dressing:
- 2 tbsp. red wine vinegar
- 4 tablespoons olive oil
- Freshly ground black pepper
- 3/4 cup finely coarsely ground cashews
- Sea salt

Directions:
1. Combine all of the dressing ingredients in a food processor.
2. Toss with the rest of the ingredients and combine well.

Beetroot Kalamata Olives and Artichoke Heart Salad

Ingredients:
- 2 beetroots, peeled and sliced lengthwise
- 1/2 cup Kalamata olives
- 1/2 cup artichoke hearts

Dressing:
- 2 tbsp. white wine vinegar
- 4 tablespoons extra virgin olive oil
- Freshly ground black pepper
- 3/4 cup finely ground almonds
- Sea salt

Directions:
1. Combine all of the dressing ingredients in a food processor.
2. Toss with the rest of the ingredients and combine well.

Boston Lettuce Baby Carrots and Artichoke Heart Salad

Ingredients:
- 1 head Boston lettuce, rinsed, patted and shredded
- 1/2 baby carrots
- 1/2 cup artichoke hearts

Dressing:
- 2 tbsp. white wine vinegar
- 4 tablespoons extra virgin olive oil
- Freshly ground black pepper
- 3/4 cup finely ground peanuts
- **Sea salt**

Directions:
1. Combine all of the dressing ingredients in a food processor.
2. Toss with the rest of the ingredients and combine well.

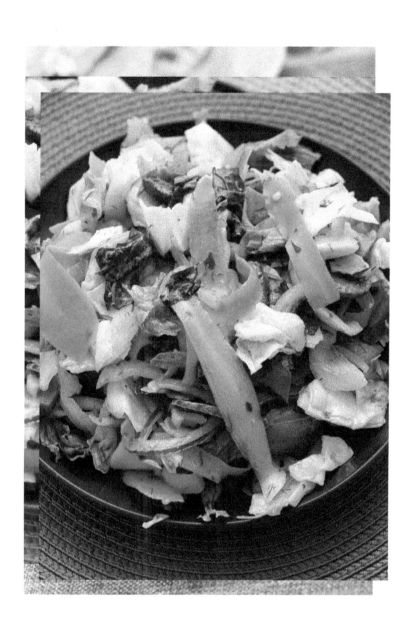

Romaine Lettuce & Baby Carrots with Walnut Vinaigrette Salad

Ingredients:
- 1 bunch of kale, rinsed, patted and shredded
- 1/2 cup black olives
- 1/2 cup baby carrots

Dressing:
- 2 tbsp. white wine vinegar
- 4 tablespoons extra virgin olive oil
- Freshly ground black pepper
- 3/4 cup finely coarsely ground walnuts
- Sea salt

Directions:
1. Combine all of the dressing ingredients in a food processor.
2. Toss with the rest of the ingredients and combine well.

Romaine Lettuce Green Olives and Artichoke Heart with Macadamia Vinaigrette

Ingredients:
- 1 head Boston lettuce, rinsed, patted and shredded
- 1/2 cup green olives
- 1/2cup artichoke hearts

Dressing:
- 2 tbsp. balsamic vinegar
- 4 tablespoons macadamia oil
- Freshly ground black pepper
- 3/4 cup finely coarsely ground cashews
- Sea salt

Directions:
1. Combine all of the dressing ingredients in a food processor.
2. Toss with the rest of the ingredients and combine well.

Collard Greens with Baby Corn Salad

Ingredients:
- 1 bunch of collard greens
- 1/2 cup black olives
- 1/2 cup canned baby corn

Dressing:
- 2 tbsp. red wine vinegar
- 4 tablespoons extra virgin olive oil
- Freshly ground black pepper
- 3/4 cup finely ground almonds
- Sea salt

Directions:
1. Combine all of the dressing ingredients in a food processor. Toss with the rest of the ingredients and combine well.

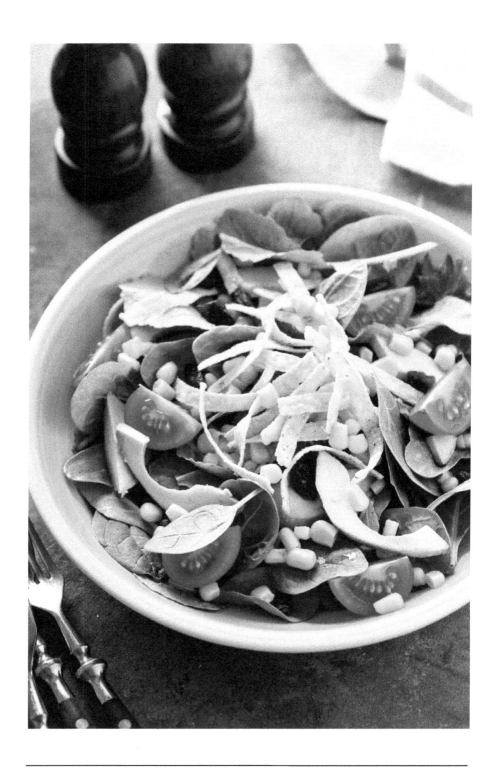

Bib Lettuce Black Olives and Baby Corn with Almond Vinaigrette Salad

Ingredients:
- 1 head Bib lettuce, rinsed, patted and shredded
- 1/2 cup black olives
- 1/2 cup canned baby corn

Dressing:
- 2 tbsp. white wine vinegar
- 4 tablespoons olive oil
- Freshly ground black pepper
- 3/4 cup finely ground almonds
- Sea salt

Directions:
1. Combine all of the dressing ingredients in a food processor.
2. Toss with the rest of the ingredients and combine well.

Mixed Greens Olives and Artichoke Heart Salad

Ingredients:
- 1 bunch of mixed greens, rinsed, patted and shredded
- 1/2 cup black olives
- 1/2 cup artichoke hearts

Dressing:
- 2 tbsp. white wine vinegar
- 4 tablespoons extra virgin olive oil
- Freshly ground black pepper
- 3/4 cup finely coarsely ground walnuts
- Sea salt

Directions:
1. Combine all of the dressing ingredients in a food processor.
2. Toss with the rest of the ingredients and combine well.

Artichoke Capers and Artichoke Heart Salad

Ingredients:
- 1 artichoke, rinsed, patted and shredded
- 1/2 cup capers
- 1/2 cup artichoke hearts

Dressing:
- 2 tbsp. white wine vinegar
- 4 tablespoons extra virgin olive oil
- Freshly ground black pepper
- 3/4 cup finely ground almonds
- Sea salt

Directions:
1. Combine all of the dressing ingredients in a food processor.
2. Toss with the rest of the ingredients and combine well.

Bibb Lettuce with Tomatillo Dressing

Ingredients:
- 1 head Bib lettuce, shredded
- 4 large tomatoes, seeded and chopped
- 4 radishes, thinly sliced

Dressing:
- 6 tomatillos, rinsed and halved
- 1 jalapeno, halved
- 1 white onion, quartered
- 2 tablespoons extra virgin olive oil
- Kosher salt and freshly ground black pepper
- 1/2 teaspoon ground cumin
- 1 cup Dairy free cream cheese
- 2 tablespoons fresh lemon juice

Directions:
1. Preheat the oven to 400 degrees F.
2. For the dressing, place the tomatillos, jalapeno and onion on a cookie sheet.
3. Drizzle with olive oil and sprinkle with salt and pepper.
4. Roast in the oven for 25- 30 min. until vegetables begin to brown and slightly darken.
5. Transfer to a food processor and let it cool then blend.

6. Add the rest of the ingredients and refrigerate for an hour.
7. Toss with the rest of the ingredients and combine well.

Plum Tomato Cucumber and Ricotta Salad

Ingredients:
- 5 medium plum tomatoes, halved lengthwise, seeded, and thinly sliced
- 1/4 white onion, peeled, halved lengthwise, and thinly sliced
- 1 large cucumber, halved lengthwise and thinly sliced
- 5 ounces ricotta cheese

Dressing:
- 1/4cup extra-virgin olive oil
- 2 splashes white wine vinegar
- Coarse salt and black pepper

Directions:
1. Combine all of the dressing ingredients.
2. Toss with the rest of the ingredients and combine well.

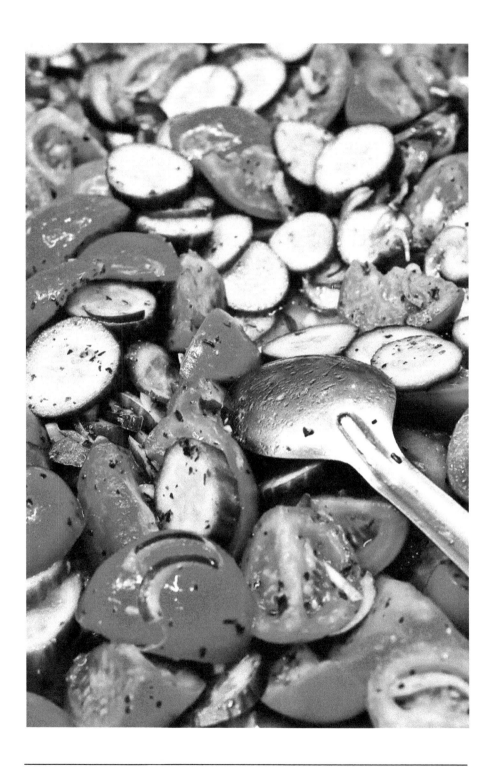

Notes

Lightning Source UK Ltd.
Milton Keynes UK
UKHW020815250521
384336UK00004B/167